MARTHA ROGERS

Notes on Nursing Theories

SERIES EDITORS

Chris Metzger McQuiston
Doctoral Candidate, Wayne State University

Adele A. Webb
College of Nursing, University of Akron

Notes on Nursing Theories is a series of monographs designed to provide the reader with a concise description of conceptual frameworks and theories in nursing. Each monograph includes a biographical sketch of the theorist, origin of the theory, assumptions, concepts, propositions, examples for application to practice and research, a glossary of terms, and a bibliography of classic works, critiques, and research.

All monographs are available for individual purchase.

MARTHA ROGERS

The Science of Unitary Human Beings

Louette R. Johnson Lutjens

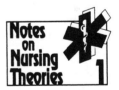

Notes on Nursing Theories 1

SAGE PUBLICATIONS
The International Professional Publishers
Newbury Park   London   New Delhi

For information address:

 SAGE Publications, Inc.
2455 Teller Road
Newbury Park, California 91320
E-mail: order@sagepub.com

SAGE Publications Ltd.
6 Bonhill Street
London EC2A 4PU
United Kingdom

SAGE Publications India Pvt. Ltd.
M-32 Market
Greater Kailash I
New Delhi 110 048 India

Printed in the United States of America

Library of Congress Cataloging-in-Publication Data

Lutjens, Louette R. Johnson.
  Martha Rogers : the science of unitary human beings / Louette R. Johnson Lutjens.
      p. cm. —(Notes on nursing theories ; v. 1)
  Includes bibliographical references.
  ISBN 0-8039-4578-7 (cl) ISBN 0-8039-4229-X (pb)
  1. Nursing—Philosophy. I. Title. II. Series: Notes on nursing theories ; vol. 1.
RT84.5.L89 1991
610.73'01—dc20   91-27264
                                                                      CIP

97 98 99 00 01 02 9 8 7 6 5

Sage Production Editor: Michelle R. Starika

To my husband,
Larry R. Lutjens, and
my children,
Chad and Heidi Lynn Lutjens

Contents

Foreword

Conceptual models are representations of the universe; therefore, one's perception of reality relates to the particular model used. Rogers's Science of Unitary Human Beings is a particular lens with which to view the universe, whereby a reality is created that requires specific beliefs about the relationships of human beings and their environments. The broad generalizations of the Science of Unitary Human Beings enable nurses to peer into the wholeness of the universe and to be creative and imaginative in their participation in the emerging science of wholeness.

The Science of Unitary Human Beings presents a framework for the construction of theories to understand the pattern of the wholeness of reality. The broad generalizations and theories guide perceptions in the way people think and what they look for in phenomena and their relationships. Through such a process, nursing science advances through the generation of *nursing* knowledge. This knowledge of the wholeness of human beings is necessary to help people participate knowingly in unfolding their potentials.

This monograph is a tribute to Martha E. Rogers. It whets one's appetite to go to her original writings to comprehend the details of her prophetic vision, especially how it participated in the shaping of the science of nursing. The author accomplishes this through a succinct presentation that synthesizes the major ideas in Rogers's writings.

The author swiftly leads the reader along a path of enlightenment of Rogers's science through concise writing. This intellectual journey includes the current thinking of Rogers, where effective use of figures and tables highlights major structural characteristics. The importance of this journey is recognized through demonstrating that nursing is concerned with the *to know* rather than just the *to do*, signifying that a scientific body of knowledge is required.

A specific example illustrates the use of the Science of Unitary Human Beings in a clinical situation, where the enigma of health is clarified from a Rogerian perspective. Rogers's futuristic perspectives are synthesized to illustrate how health and human potentials need to be viewed differently.

The unfolding of Rogers's science does not end, but continues in her theories. The author shows briefly that the thoughts and paths of other nurse theorists have as their wellspring Rogers's Science of Unitary Human Beings.

This monograph is a testament that nurses in the future will resonate with the rhythms of Rogers's vision. Rogerian scholars will have the joy of being the "hundredth monkey" in the advancement of nursing science within a science of wholeness.

JOHN R. PHILLIPS, RN, PHD
Associate Professor,
Division of Nursing,
School of Education, Health,
Nursing, and Arts Professions,
New York University

Preface

Dr. Martha E. Rogers presented an evolutionary model of humans in *An Introduction to the Theoretical Basis of Nursing* (1970). Her view of nursing as a science of unitary human beings pioneered a radical shift in thinking within the profession.

The Science of Unitary Human Beings challenges traditional ways of thinking about the world and about nursing. This new world view, characterized by energy fields, continuous mutual change in humans and their environment, no causality, and a reality unbounded by space and time, is called an abstract system by Rogers. This abstract system is science and not to be confused with the more commonly used terms of conceptual model or theory (Rogers, personal communication, November 11, 1990). The terms used in the Science of Unitary Human Beings are unique to the abstract system. The two common reactions of students to this abstract system are either one of immediate bonding with Rogers's way of thinking or one of disregard because her science is viewed as too abstract to be useful in nursing practice. Most would agree that the ideas put forth by Martha Rogers are exciting.

There are many nurse scholars who conduct research and practice based on Rogers's abstract system. They have formed the Society of Rogerian Scholars, which holds conferences and publishes the *Rogerian Nursing Science Newsletter*. Also, many doctoral students at New York University (where Rogers is Professor Emerita) and other universities in the United States and other countries use the Science of Unitary Human Beings for their dissertation research. This science also serves as the basis for programs in nursing education and practice and administrative decision-making in nursing service.

Martha Rogers, as one of the foremost thinkers in nursing today, serves as an inspiration to faculty as well as students. She continues to develop her science based on research and new thinking. The evolutionary nature of her abstract system is apropos to a view of humans as forever changing and evolving. The ongoing development of the Science of Unitary Human Beings challenges students of nursing theory to keep current. Examples of the continuing development of this science are described throughout this volume.

In her early writings, Rogers used the term *man;* thus quotes from her writings prior to 1983 use the term *man* rather than *human beings.* The change in words was an update to reflect sensitivity to the goal of gender-free language.

This volume presents a current, succinct description of Rogers's abstract system. The objective of this description is a basic understanding of a nontraditional world view, and the role of the nurse based on that world view. Serving as a summary of the abstract system, this volume supplements original sources, most recently a chapter in Barrett's book (1990). Moreover, the latest thinking of Dr. Rogers, which was gleaned from conversations between Dr. Rogers and the author in November 1990, is incorporated herein.

This volume is intended primarily for undergraduate students who are studying several conceptual models, theories, and the Science of Unitary Human Beings with their differing terms, language, and specific definitions of common concepts. It also could be used as a review by nurse faculty and graduate students.

Although several theories have been generated from this abstract system, they will not be addressed herein. The abstract nature and/or scope of these theories demand individual attention.

A bibliography is provided to direct readers to appropriate sources for in-depth information on the Rogers abstract system, theories derived from this science, nursing practice based on this abstract system, applications to practice and education, and analysis and critique of the abstract system. It is hoped that this description of Rogers's Science of Unitary Human Beings will entice readers to make use of the references provided in the bibliography.

I would like to acknowledge the careful and thoughtful critique of this volume by Dr. Barbara Girardin of California State University, San Diego, California. Special thanks also to Dr. Martha Rogers for her review and comments on an earlier draft. She is indeed inspirational.

—LOUETTE R. JOHNSON LUTJENS

Biographical Sketch of a Scientist in Nursing: Martha E. Rogers, ScD, RN, FAAN

Born: May 12, 1914, Dallas, TX
Diploma: Knoxville General Hospital School of Nursing, TN, 1936
BS: Public Health Nursing, George Peabody College, TN, 1937
MA: Teacher's College, Columbia University, NY, 1945
MPH: Johns Hopkins University, Baltimore, MD, 1952
ScD: Johns Hopkins University, Baltimore, MD, 1954
Fellow: American Academy of Nursing
Position: Professor Emerita, Division of Nursing, New York University; consultant, speaker

1

Evolution of the
Abstract System

The evolution of the Science of Unitary Human Beings began 30 years ago with the early writings of Dr. Martha E. Rogers. The development of her abstract system was strongly influenced by an early grounding in the liberal arts and an educational background in science at the University of Tennessee (1931-1933) that began two years before she entered nursing school. Her interest in space began with a fascination for air travel as a small child.

In the 1960s, Rogers advocated nursing science as unique and essential in realizing nursing's contribution to human science. For Rogers, the uniqueness of nursing as a science is its long-established concern and interest in people and their world. The Science of Unitary Human Beings was not derived from other sciences, but, rather, originated as a synthesis (not a summation) of facts and ideas from multiple sources of knowledge; a new product. The uniqueness is in the phenomena central to its concern: people and their environment. As defined in this abstract system, the uniqueness of nursing is its focus on unitary human beings and their world.

An abstract system of mutuality generates no causality (acausality). A Rogerian view of acausality emerges from an infinite universe of open systems. Cause and effect are contradictions of open systems. Similar findings, with regard to acausality, have been reported in the physical world. Specifically, these findings include Heisenberg's

3

principle of uncertainty, quantum theory, and Einstein's theory of relativity, to name but a few. Thus any words implying linear or causal relationships (e.g., cause, effect, adaptation, sequence, influence) are inconsistent with a Rogerian viewpoint. In earlier writings, Rogers used such terms as *continuum* and *unidirectional*. These linear words have been deleted in later writings to correct earlier misinterpretations. The Science of Unitary Human Beings provides a world view of a universe that is beyond our current understanding or familiarity. It includes possibilities for the future and recognizes change as basic to existence. The aim of the Science of Unitary Human Beings is to advance nursing as a learned profession, both the science and art of nursing (Rogers, 1990). As a learned profession, the art and science of nursing could be empowered to provide compassionate service to humankind now and "spacekind" in the future. The purpose of nurses is "to promote health and well-being for all persons and groups wherever they are" (Rogers, personal communication, November 11, 1990). (A Rogerian view of health will be discussed later.)

Rogers identifies and uses the word *nursing* as a noun, a learned profession. This new view differs from the traditional use of nursing as a verb or action word. Rogers's abstract system of Science of Unitary Human Beings, which was formally proposed in 1970, established her as a vanguard of a new view and vision of nursing. Her futuristic perspective is unrivaled.

Assumptions

Assumptions are givens—statements assumed to be true without proof. In *An Introduction to the Theoretical Basis of Nursing* (1970), Rogers put forth five assumptions that underlie her science of nursing. However, it must be recognized that this book was published more than 20 years ago, and that the Science of Unitary Human Beings has developed substantially over the past 20 years based on research and new thinking. Therefore, the 1970 book contains terms and language that have been replaced with terminology consistent with emerging knowledge and the development of Rogerian science (Rogers, personal communication, November 11, 1990). However, *An Introduction to the Theoretical Basis of Nursing* is considered a seminal text of historical significance. It put forth a new world view of nursing as a discipline by declaring it a science.

2

Building Blocks
of the Abstract System

As Rogers worked on the development of her abstract system, it became necessary that she become more specific. Energy fields, openness, pandimensionality, and pattern have been identified as building blocks of her abstract system (Table 2.1). These building blocks, which correspond to contemporary knowledge, have been used to develop a language of specificity for the Science of Unitary Human Beings. This science was developed to address nursing's long-held concern with persons and their environment, specifically their health.

At the time of the initial development of the Science of Unitary Human Beings, systems theory was among the many schools of thought that had a bearing on general thinking, the major features of that model being the system (unitary human being) and its environment in a mutual process that is active and dynamic. Rogers refers to a universe of open systems, and her view of systems proposes a mutual process of change in human beings and environment that is continuous. Human beings and their environments are defined as energy fields.

TABLE 2.1 The Building Blocks of the Abstract System

Energy Fields
Openness
Pandimensionality
Pattern

Energy Fields

Energy fields are "the fundamental units of the living and the non-living" (Rogers, 1990, p. 7). This is a notion that is different for those who learned that the cell was the fundamental unit of living systems, such as human beings. Field is the concept that unites humans and their environments. Energy signifies the dynamism of the human and environmental fields. Fields are infinite, in continuous motion, and always changing mutually; in essence, they are without boundaries.

Person. According to Rogers, people and their environments are the phenomena central to the focus of nursing. Human beings are wholes, not merely collections of body parts (heart, lungs) or body systems (cardiovascular, neurological). Wholeness is irreducible.

The notion of wholeness is becoming more commonplace. Recently, an exhibition of Monet serial paintings was held at art institutes across the United States. Guided tours were available on audiotapes. At one point the narrator advised patrons to stand back from the individual paintings and look at the series as a whole. This would provide a perspective of the series collection as a whole that was different than the sum of the individual paintings. Rogers's human energy fields, viewed as a whole, provide a perspective that is also irreducible and indivisible, manifesting characteristics specific to the whole. A Rogerian would not discuss or study a part of a human being since doing so would be a contradiction of wholeness.

Human beings have "the capacity for abstraction and imagery, language and thought, sensation and emotion" (Rogers, 1970, p. 73). They have the ability to perceive the universe and wonder about it. Unique human energy fields are differentiated by pattern just as fingerprints or voice prints are unique to individuals.

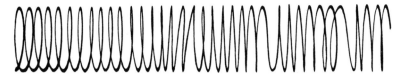

Figure 2.1. Rogers used a Slinky to illustrate the openness and rhythmical nature of the life process.
NOTE: Slinky,® James Industries Inc., Hollidayburg, PA. Used by permission.

Environment. The environmental field is also a whole with its own identity, and is also irreducible, indivisible, and differentiated by pattern. Human and environmental energy fields are integral with one another. The mutual process of the energy fields is observed in manifestations of pattern. Martha Rogers uses the analogy of an overlay to help others understand the integrality of the fields (Rogers, personal communication, November 11, 1990). When a transparent image is laid over another image the two images are united and thus integral.

Openness

The integrality of human and environmental energy fields is possible because both are open systems. Openness between human beings and their environment is continuous—that is, they are *always* open. Energy is in continuous movement. In *An Introduction to the Theoretical Basis of Nursing,* Rogers used a Slinky as a symbol of openness and the rhythmical nature of the life process (Figure 2.1). She used the Slinky initially as an aid to thinking. Although she no longer sees a need to use a Slinky to illustrate her point (Rogers, 1990), it is a useful symbol for students learning the Science of Unitary Human Beings.

Human and environmental energy fields evolve and continuously change at the same time. Through the continuous process of humans and their environment, people are different today than they were yesterday. Therefore, human beings can *never* go back. One never walks the same stream twice. The person is different and so is the stream (Rogers, Doyle, Racolin, & Walsh, 1990). Human beings do not adapt to their environment; they are integral with their environment. For that reason, the environment cannot cause something to happen to humans. "Causality is a contradiction of open systems" (Rogers, 1988, p. 100). Rogers asserted (personal communication, November 11, 1990) that adaptation, causality, equilibrium, homeostasis, and similar terms have been outmoded since the 1950s because they are unsupported in a universe of open systems.

Pandimensionality

Human beings are unique energy fields that cannot be divided or reduced. The human field is integral with its unique environmental field, which also cannot be divided or reduced. Both fields have infinite dimensions. Because we live in a three-dimensional reality, we understand it, but that does not mean that there are no other realities. We have limited our thinking to the traditional three-dimensional world view. In earlier writings, Rogers used the term *four-dimensionality* to define a reality without spatial or temporal attributes. As her abstract system continued to develop, it became increasingly clear that four-dimensionality was not consistent with the definition that had emerged, and multidimensionality (Rogers, 1990) was substituted for four-dimensionality for a brief time. These two terms are now viewed as misnomers and have been replaced by *pandimensionality*, which better corresponds with the definition of a nonlinear domain without spatial and temporal attributes. The term refers to a reality that is different than a three-dimensional world view. Pandimensionality is a new reality, a way of perceiving that is a new and different way to view the world. Paranormal events, such as deja vu, clairvoyance, and other phenomena, can be explained with Rogers's view of pandimensional reality, unique human energy fields united with their unique environment in an infinite domain.

Pattern

Human energy fields can be differentiated from their environmental energy fields by pattern. Pattern is an abstraction that cannot be seen; however, manifestations of a pattern can be observed. The pattern is in the form of a single wave. Field patterns demonstrate increasing variation and continual change. Therefore, the field patterns are unpredictable, dynamic, creative, and continuously innovative.

Manifestions of pattern unite humans and environments in the variations in their patterns. They represent expressions of the unique relationship of individual human beings and their environment. Manifestations of patterns can be observed in a manner similar to looking into a kaleidoscope to see continually changing patterns brought about by unique relationships among bits of colored glass and reflecting surfaces. As the instrument is rotated, similar to the passage of time, there is constant change, continuous variations in form, revealing new, creative, and innovative manifestations of pattern. Some of the changes are subtle, but the observed patterns are *never* the same. There is order to the display, but it contains variations, differences, and a uniqueness with each rotation of the kaleidoscope.

In humans, patterns are abstractions that display themselves as nonrepeating rhythms in human behavior, such as sleep and waking and perceptions of time and motion. In Rogers's earlier writings, the manifestations of field patterning were called correlates. Pattern manifestation signifies mutual process of human and environmental energy fields. This process occurs continually in infinite dimensions. Manifestations of the diversity in field patterning can be seen in, for example, perceptions of time. One person may experience a day as very long, while another may talk about how the day just flew by. It is not uncommon for a person to think that it takes longer to get someplace than to come home from that place though the distance is the same. It should be clear that the evidence or manifestation of human field patterns is specific to the whole person, not just to one of the parts. For example, as Rogers's abstract system clarifies nursing, it would be inappropriate to treat only a part of the whole person such as the cardiovascular system of a patient. However, you could facilitate comfort during chest pain with guided imagery and observe the change in the duration of chest pain. Rogers views human bodies as manifestations of field. This view of humans and the purpose of nurses is distinct to Rogers's abstract system.

Nursing is also concerned with groups. Two or more people constitute a group, which is its own energy field, integral with its own unique environmental field. Nurses must decide whether they are going to focus on a group energy field, such as family, community, or mother/baby dyad, or an individual energy field, such as family member, community member, mother, or baby (Rogers, 1990). Group energy fields, like human energy fields, are irreducible and indivisible. Therefore, information about group members does not provide information about the group or vice versa. In other words, one cannot generalize from a part (individual group member) to a whole (group). The focus of nursing on human beings and their world as wholes as defined by the Science of Unitary Human Beings is unique to nursing.

3

Nursing

Nursing is a learned profession—that is, it is a science and an art (Rogers, 1990). "Nursing is the study of unitary, irreducible, indivisible human and environmental [energy] fields" (Rogers, p. 6). It is an organized body of abstract knowledge about people and their world. The art of nursing involves the imaginative and creative use of nursing knowledge (science). The purpose of nurses is to promote health and well-being for all persons and groups wherever they are using the art and science of nursing. Rogers emphasizes that health (versus sickness) services should be community based. Sickness services are traditional to health care settings. Thus Rogers challenges nurses to consider the nursing needs of all people, including future generations of spacekind, as life continues to evolve from earth to space and beyond. The Science of Unitary Human Beings provides a different world view that encompasses a practice of nursing for the present time and for the imagined and yet-to-be imagined future. Rogers envisions a nursing practice of noninvasive modalities, such as therapeutic touch (Krieger, 1979; Quinn, 1989), humor, guided imagery (Butcher & Parker, 1988), use of color, light (Girardin, 1990), music, and meditation focusing on the health potential of the person.

4

Principles of Homeodynamics

The Science of Unitary Human Beings has generated three principles of homeodynamics that provide a foundation for nursing practice: integrality, resonancy and helicy (Table 4.1). These principles provide "fundamental guides to the practice of nursing" (Rogers, 1990, p. 8). The four building blocks (energy field, openness, pandimensionality, pattern) previously described are evident in the principles of Rogers's science and propose a view of change as evolutionary. All of the principles of homeodynamics are characterized by continuous change.

Integrality

The principle of integrality states that human and environmental fields are a continuous and mutual process. The two fields are open systems integral with one another. Use of such terms as simultaneous, changing together, and exchange, to name a few, would be incongruent with the principle of integrality because they imply separateness rather than unity.

The continuous mutual flow of energy of human beings and their environments creates constant changes in the life process. Human beings and their environments are continually being identified by different manifestations (Rogers, 1970). As the mountain climber ascends to higher altitudes, continuous changes occur from the dynamic

TABLE 4.1 Principles of Homeodynamics

Integrality
Resonancy
Helicy

mutual process of the human and the environment. Thus the change in altitude does not *cause* changes in the climber, nor does the climber *adapt* to the altitude. The principle of integrality firmly rejects the idea of causality.

Resonancy

The principle of resonancy asserts that manifestations of patterns characterizing human and environmental energy fields are continuously changing from lower frequency, longer waves to higher frequency, shorter waves. The life process in human beings is a symphony of rhythmical vibrations that gives intensity to the life process. The life process becomes increasingly diverse. There are more variations, greater differences. Each turn of the spiral in the Slinky (see Figure 2.1) symbolizes the rhythmical nature of life. Human beings experience their environment by resonating patterns.

Helicy

The principle of helicy tells us that human and environmental field patterns are continuous, innovative, unpredictable, and increasing in diversity. In 1990, Rogers substituted the word *unpredictable* for *probabilistic*. The deletion of probability in favor of unpredictability was associated with the emergence of chaos theory discussed in the recent works of such authors as Mallove, and Peterson, as well as others. The change to unpredictability "strengthens consistency and supports the nature of change proposed in the principles of homeodynamics" (Rogers, 1990, p. 7).

The life process is evolutionary in that constant change is taking place that draws upon the past. Through continuous change, new, nonrepeating rhythmical patterns continue to emerge, becoming more diverse, possessing more variation, and becoming unpredictable. This is *becoming*.

Nursing practice chiefly involves assessment and identification of the manifestations of patterns that emerge from the mutual person and environmental energy field process and deliberative patterning through a nurse and person mutual process. The nurse's energy field and the person's energy field together participate in patterning toward optimum health potential. Unique and constantly changing human and environmental field patterns require nursing interventions that are different for each person. Through its practice, nursing seeks to promote harmony of human and environmental energy fields, to strengthen coherence and integrity of human fields, and to participate in direct and redirect patterning of human and environmental energy fields toward the goal of optimum health potential (Rogers, 1970). An excellent example of nursing practice with a focus on patterning can be found in Madrid (1990).

5

Clinical Example

Madrid (1990) recounts a clinical experience with a young man hospitalized for gastrointestinal bleeding secondary to Acquired Immune Deficiency Syndrome (AIDS), providing a view of the transformation of this man, manifesting patterns of energy depletion, pain, and restlessness to patterns of peace, enjoyment, and interest in self and his environment. The transformation occurs through the process of mutual (person and nurse) patterning of the self and environment using Rogerian practice modalities.

Madrid used imagination and imagery to achieve a picture of what this man's life was like before he became ill. These techniques enabled her to experience a richer perception of him as a unitary human being that transcended his present ill health. She promoted comfort through deep breathing, relaxation exercises, and therapeutic touch. Music was used to achieve a sense of peace, and guided imagery was utilized to capture enjoyable moments from the past. Also, her *presence* as a nurse was used as a therapeutic modality to promote comfort. Throughout this experience, Madrid used Rogerian practice methodology of pattern manifestation appraisal and deliberative mutual patterning involving the nurse and the sick person's energy fields in mutual process.

6

Health

Rogers does not give an explicit definition of health. She considers it an ambiguous term that is used in many different ways. She states that both health and sickness are expressions of the life process and are determined by individuals and cultures; therefore, they are value-laden words. Contemporary major American health problems are iatrogenesis (induced by physicians), nosocomial (induced by hospitals) infections, and nosophobia (fear of disease) according to Rogers (1990, p. 5). Behaviors of low value to an individual or culture may be labeled *sick*, whereas behaviors of high value may be labeled *health*. Some values change over time. At one time homosexuality was generally considered a sick behavior, a behavioral disease, in the United States. Persons exhibiting such behavior were hospitalized in psychiatric units, and great effort was extended to change their homosexual behavior to heterosexual behavior. Rogers seems to prefer the term *human betterment* over health because the former is less ambiguous. Having a diagnosis, a label, is sometimes enough to cripple action (e.g., cardiac cripples). Also, Rogers does not use the term *patient*. She considers the term too restrictive. The word patient does not encompass the majority of people, and people are nursing's concern (Rogers, personal communication, November 11, 1990).

From a futuristic perspective, Rogers explains that what is disease or sickness today may not be pathological in the future (Rogers, 1990). Current physiological parameters of a normal hemoglobin or pulmonary vital capacity may not hold for future generations. Loss of calcium has been observed in astronauts; perhaps, spacekind will not need the amount of calcium required by humankind. Rogers believes a new species will emerge: spacekind. "Homo spacialis" will evolve and transcend homo sapiens. The normal parameters for the great grandchildren of the young adults of today that will be residing in a space station in the year 2050 may be entirely different from those of their great grandparents residing on earth. Humankind will change and evolve continuously and mutually with its environments to spacekind and beyond.

Future health services are predicted to be community based, with an orientation to health, as contrasted with what now might better be called hospital or sickness orientation. Health promotion rather than cure of disease will be the focus. The practice of nursing will be identified through noninvasive modalities with a purpose of promoting human betterment.

7

Related Theories

A science generates many theories. Among the theories proposed by Rogers, three have received the most attention in the literature: accelerating change, paranormal phenomena, and rhythmical manifestations of change.

The theory of accelerating change holds that change is speeding up and that there is greater diversity of human and environmental fields. This theory provides an explanation for the hyperactivity observed more frequently in children today.

The theory of paranormal phenomena provides an explanation for precognition, deja vu, clairvoyance, and telepathy. In a pandimensional world, there are no limits imposed by space and time. Human and environmental fields are integral. Therefore, the present is relative to the person.

"The theory of rhythmical [manifestations] of change focuses on human and environmental field rhythms" (Fawcett, 1989, p. 278). This theory deals with manifestations of human and environmental field patterns, such as sleep/wake patterns (Floyd, 1983) and perceptions of time passing (Fitzpatrick, Donovan, & Johnston, 1980), to name but a few manifestations.

The Science of Unitary Human Beings was foundational for the development of some theories of nursing. These theories are in varying stages of development. One example is Margaret Newman's Model of Health as an Expansion of Consciousness (1986). The focus of her theory is the nature of health. The three definitions of health proposed by Newman (expanding consciousness, disease-nondisease fusion, person and environment) have pattern as a common element. Additionally, the concepts of consciousness, movement, time, and space with which Newman views health reflect the influence of Rogers.

Rosemarie Rizzo Parse's Man-Living-Health model (1981) is considered Rogerian science that has been modified to include existential phenomenological thought. The focus of Parse's theory is the meaning underlying the behavior of human beings as they relate with the environment.

Rogerian scholars conduct basic and applied research using the Science of Unitary Human Beings. Basic research is theoretical research that extends the base of knowledge for the sake of knowledge itself. An example is Barrett's theory of power (Barrett, 1990), which was derived from Rogers's principle of helicy. "Power is defined as the capacity to participate knowingly in the nature of change characterizing the continuous patterning of the human and environmental fields as manifest by awareness, choices, freedom to act intentionally, and involvement in creating change" (p. 108). The concepts of awareness, choices, freedom to act intentionally, and involvement in creating change were used as empirical indicators of power to test the hypothesis that power was related to human field motion (Barrett, 1990). Barrett developed an instrument, the Barrett Power as Knowing Participation in Change Test, to measure field patterns of power.

Another example of applied research using the Science of Unitary Human Beings is Ference's research in human field motion. A theory of motion was derived from the principle of resonancy. This theory "proposes that as a human field engages in ever-higher levels of human field motion, the pattern evolves toward greater . . . diversity and differentiation" (Ference, 1989, p. 123). The Ference Human Field Motion Tool was developed to measure evaluation of change. Ference found in her research that human field motion expanded with greater physical motion (Ference, 1989). Other researchers have found that human field motion also expands with meditation, risk-taking, and higher levels of participation in change (Ference, 1989).

Applied research seeks to find solutions to practical problems. An example of applied research using Rogerian science is Andersen's LIGHT model (Andersen & Smereck, 1989). This is a prescriptive model synthesized from Aristotle's theory of ethics and the Science of Unitary Human Beings. The Personalized Nursing LIGHT model has two tracks. One track, personalized care, consists of all actions taken by a nurse on behalf of persons with the intent of improving their well-being. The other track, personalized action, consists of all actions taken by the person to achieve well-being. "Both tracks are described with the acronym LIGHT" (p. 122). The Personalized Nursing LIGHT Model" has been implemented successfully with patients confined to a psychiatric institution, with persons treated in a mental health nursing clinic, and with persons who are intravenous drug abusers in urban community outreach programs in three states" (p. 120).

Martha Rogers continues to have a profound influence on nursing as a profession and as a science. Rogerian scholars believe the Science of Unitary Human Beings is *the* nursing science. They constitute probably the best organized band of theory scholars of any of the nurse theorists. These scholars are developing an ever-widening program of research to clarify, expand and extend understanding of the Science of Unitary Human Beings. Even those who do not promote Rogers's abstract system recognize that Martha E. Rogers has challenged traditional ways of thinking and encouraged futuristic thinking. More importantly, she has identified what is unique to nursing.

Glossary

Building Blocks

Energy field
"The fundamental unit of the living and the non-living. Field is a unifying concept. Energy signifies the dynamic nature of the field; a field is in continuous motion and is infinite" (Rogers, 1990, p. 7).

Environmental field (environment)
"An irreducible, indivisible, pandimensional energy field identified by pattern and integral with the human field" (Rogers, 1990, p. 7).

Four-dimensionality
Retitled pandimensionality (Rogers, personal communication, November, 11, 1990).

Human field
See *unitary human beings*.

Pandimensionality
"A nonlinear domain without spatial or temporal attributes...provides for an infinite domain without limit" (Rogers, 1990, p. 7). Formerly titled four-dimensionality and multidimensionality.

Pattern
"The distinguishing characteristic of an energy field perceived as a single wave" (Rogers, 1990, p. 7).

Unitary human beings (human field)

"An irreducible, indivisible, pandimensional energy field identified by pattern and manifesting characteristics that are specific to the whole and which cannot be predicted from knowledge of the parts" (Rogers, 1990, p. 7).

Principles of Homeodynamics

"Provide fundamental guides to the practice of nursing" (Rogers, 1990, p. 8).

Helicy

"Continuous, innovative, unpredictable, increasing diversity of human and environmental field patterns" (Rogers, 1990, p. 8).

Integrality

"Continuous mutual human field and environmental field process" (Rogers, 1990, p. 8). Formerly titled complementarity.

Resonancy

"Continuous change from lower to higher frequency wave patterns in human and environmental fields" (Rogers, 1990, p. 8).

Related Terms

Health

"Unitary human health signifies an irreducible human field manifestation" (Rogers, 1990, p. 10); human betterment (Rogers, 1990, p. 10); an expression "of the process of life" (Rogers, 1970, p. 85); a value defined by individuals and cultures.

Nursing

"Learned profession"; "a science and an art" (Rogers, 1990, p. 5); a basic science (Rogers, personal communication, November 11, 1990); "study of unitary, irreducible, indivisible human and environmental fields: people and their world (Rogers, 1990, p. 6).

Art of nursing: "Creative use of the science of nursing for human betterment" (Rogers, 1990, p. 6); imaginative and creative use of nursing knowledge (Rogers, 1990, p. 387).

Purpose of nurses: "Promote health and well being for all persons and groups wherever they are" (Rogers, personal communication, November, 11, 1990).

Uniqueness of nursing: The "focus on unitary human beings and their world" (Rogers, 1990, p. 6).

Science
"An organized body of abstract knowledge" (Rogers, personal communication, November 11, 1990); "a synthesis of facts and ideas; a new product" (Rogers, 1990, p. 6).

References

Andersen, M., & Smereck, G. A. D. (1989). Personalized nursing LIGHT model. *Nursing Science Quarterly, 2,* 120-130.

Barrett, E. A. M. (1990). Health patterning with clients in a private practice environment. In E. A. M. Barrett (Ed.), *Visions of Rogers' science-based nursing* (pp. 105-115). New York: National League for Nursing Pub. No. 15-2285.

Butcher, H. R., & Parker, N. I. (1988). Guided imagery within Rogers' science of unitary human beings: An experimental study. *Nursing Science Quarterly, 1,* 103-110.

Fawcett, J. (1989). *Analysis and evaluation of conceptual models of nursing* (2nd ed., pp. 263-305). Philadelphia: F. A. Davis.

Ference, H. M. (1989). Nursing science theories and administration. In B. Henry, C. Arndt, M. Di Vincenti, & A. Marriner-Tomey, *Dimensions of nursing administration: Theory, research, education, practice* (pp. 121-131). Boston: Blackwell Scientific.

Fitzpatrick, J. J., Donovan, M. J., & Johnston, R. L. (1980). Experience of time during the crisis of cancer. *Cancer Nursing, 3,* 191-194.

Floyd, J. (1983). Research using Rogers' conceptual system: Development of a testable theorem. *Advances in Nursing Science, 5*(2), 37-48.

Girardin, B. (1990). *The relationship of light wave frequency and sleepwakefulness frequency in well, full-term Hispanic neonates.* Unpublished doctoral dissertation, Wayne State University, Detroit.

Krieger, D. (1979). *Therapeutic touch: How to use your hands to help and heal.* Englewood Cliffs, NJ: Prentice-Hall.

Madrid, M. (1990). The participating process of human field patterning in an acute-care environment. In E. A. M. Barrett (Ed.), *Visions of Rogers' science-based nursing* (pp. 93-104). New York: National League for Nursing Pub. No. 15-2285.

Newman, M. (1986). *Health as expanding consciousness.* St. Louis: C.V. Mosby.

Parse, R. R. (1981). *Man-living-health: A theory of nursing.* New York: Wiley.

Quinn, J. F. (1989). Therapeutic touch as energy exchange: Replication and extension. *Nursing Science Quarterly, 2,* 79-87.

Rogers, M. E. (1970). *An introduction to the theoretical basis of nursing.* Philadelphia: F. A. Davis.

Rogers, M. E. (1988). Nursing science and art: A prospective. *Nursing Science Quarterly, 1,* 99-102.

Rogers, M. E. (1990). Nursing: Science of unitary, irreducible, human beings: Update 1990. In E. A. M. Barrett (Ed.), *Visions of Rogers' science-based nursing* (pp. 5-11). New York: National League for Nursing Pub. No. 15-2285.

Rogers, M. E., Doyle, M. B., Racolin, A., & Walsh, P. C. (1990). A conversation with Martha Rogers on nursing in space. In E. A. M. Barrett (Ed.), *Visions of Rogers' science-based nursing* (pp. 375-386). New York: National League for Nursing Pub. No. 15-2285.

Bibliography

Biography of Dr. Martha E. Rogers

Gioiella, E. (1989). Professionalizing nursing: A Rogers legacy. *Nursing Science Quarterly, 2,* 61-62.

Hektor, L. M. (1989). Martha E. Rogers: A life history. *Nursing Science Quarterly, 2,* 63-73.

Parse, R. R. (1989). Martha E. Rogers: A birthday celebration. *Nursing Science Quarterly, 2,* 55.

The Abstract System

Barrett, E. A. M. (1990). Health patterning with clients in a private practice environment. In E. A. M. Barrett (Ed.), *Visions of Rogers' science-based nursing* (Publication No. 15-2285, pp. 105-115). New York: National League for Nursing.

Chinn, P. L. & Kramer, M. K. (1991). *Theory and nursing: A systematic approach* (3rd ed., pp. 182-183). St. Louis: C. V. Mosby.

Daily, J. S., Maupin, J. S., Satterly, M. C., Schnell, D. L., & Wallace, T. L. (1989). Martha E. Rogers: Unitary human beings. In A. Marriner-Tomey (Ed.), *Nursing theorists and their work* (2nd ed., pp. 402-412). St. Louis: C. V. Mosby.

Falco, S. M., & Lobo, M. L. (1990). Martha E. Rogers. In J. B. George (Ed.), *Nursing theories: The base for professional nursing practice* (pp. 211-230). Norwalk, CT: Appleton & Lange.

Leddy, S., & Pepper, J. M. (1989). *Conceptual bases of professional nursing* (2nd ed., pp. 188-190). Philadelphia: J. B. Lippincott.

Malinkski, V. (Ed.). (1986). *Explorations on Martha Rogers' Science of Unitary Human Beings.* Norwalk, CT: Appleton & Lange.

Newman, M. (1986). *Health as expanding consciousness.* St. Louis: C. V. Mosby.

Parse, R. R. (1981). *Man-living-health: A theory of nursing.* New York: Wiley.
Rogers, M. E. (1970). *The theoretical basis of nursing.* Philadelphia: F. A. Davis.
Rogers, M. E. (1988). Nursing science and art: A prospective. *Nursing Science Quarterly, 1*, 99-102.
Rogers, M. E. (1989). Nursing: A science of unitary human beings. In J. P. Riehl-Sisca (Ed.), *Conceptual models for nursing practice* (3rd ed., pp. 181-188). Norwalk, CT: Appleton & Lange.
Rogers, M. E. (1990). Nursing: Science of unitary, irreducible, human beings: Update 1990. In E. A. M. Barrett (Ed.), *Visions of Rogers' science-based nursing* (Publication No. 15-2285, pp. 5-11). New York: National League for Nursing.
Rogers, M. E., Doyle, M. B., Racolin, A., & Walsh, P. C. (1990). A conversation with Martha Rogers on nursing in space. In E. A. M. Barrett (Ed.), *Visions of Rogers' science-based nursing* (Publication No. 15-2285, pp. 375-386). New York: National League for Nursing.
Reeder, F. (1984). Philosophic issues in the Rogerian science of unitary human beings. *Advances in Nursing Science, 6*, 14-23.
Sarter, B. (1988a). *The stream of becoming: A study of Martha Rogers's theory* (Publication No. 15-2205). New York: National League for Nursing.
Sarter, B. (1988b). Philosophical sources of nursing theory. *Nursing Science Quarterly, 1*, 52-59.
Sarter, B. (1989). Some critical philosophical issues in the science of unitary human beings. *Nursing Science Quarterly, 2*, 74-78.
Smith, M. J. (1989). Four dimensionality: Where to go with it. *Nursing Science Quarterly, 2*, 56.

Analysis and Evaluation of the Science of Unitary Human Beings

Cerilli, K., & Burd, S. (1989). An analysis of Martha Rogers' nursing as a science of unitary human beings. In J. P. Riehl-Sisca (Ed.), *Conceptual models for nursing practice* (3rd ed., pp. 189-194). Norwalk, CT: Appleton & Lange.
Fawcett, J. (1989). Rogers' science of unitary human beings. *Analysis and evaluation of conceptual models of nursing* (2nd ed., pp. 263-305). Philadelphia: F. A. Davis.
Quillin, S. I. M., & Runk, J. A. (1989). Martha Rogers' unitary person model. In J. J. Fitzpatrick & A. L. Whall (Eds.), *Conceptual model of nursing* (2nd ed., pp. 285-300). Norwalk, CT: Appleton & Lange.
Whall, A. L. (1987). A critique of Rogers's framework. In R. R. Parse (Ed.), *Major paradigms, theories and critiques* (pp. 147-158). Philadelphia: W. B. Saunders.

Extensions of the Science of Unitary Human Beings to Groups

Alligood, M. R. (1989). Rogers' theory and nursing administration: A perspective on health and environment. In B. Henry, C. Arndt, M. Di Vincenti, & A. Marriner-Tomey, *Dimensions of nursing administration: Theory, research, education, practice* (pp. 105-111). Boston: Blackwell Scientific.
Ference, H. M. (1989). Nursing science theories and administration. In B. Henry, C. Arndt, M. Di Vincenti, & A. Marriner-Tomey, *Dimensions of nursing adminis-*

28 MARTHA ROGERS

tration: Theory, research, education, practice (pp. 121-131). Boston: Blackwell Scientific.

Gueldner, S. H. (1989). Applying Rogers's model to nursing administration: Emphasis on client and nursing. In B. Henry, C. Arndt, M. Di Vincenti, & A. Marriner-Tomey, *Dimensions of nursing administration: Theory, research, education, practice* (pp. 113-119). Boston: Blackwell Scientific.

Hanchett, E. S. (1989). *Nursing frameworks and community as client: Bridging the gap.* Norwalk, CT: Appleton & Lange.

Hanchett, E. S. (1990). Nursing models and community as client. *Nursing Science Quarterly, 3,* 67-72.

Research and Applications to Practice

Alligood, M. R. (1991). Testing Rogers' theory of accelerating change: The relationships among creativity, actualization, and empathy in persons 18 to 92 years of age. *Western Journal of Nursing Research, 13*(1), 84-96.

Andersen, M. D., & Smereck, G. A. D. (1989). Personalized nursing LIGHT model. *Nursing Science Quarterly, 2,* 120-130.

Barrett, E. A. M. (1988). Using Rogers' science of unitary human beings in nursing practice. *Nursing Science Quarterly, 1,* 50-51.

Barrett, E. A. M. (Ed.). (1990a). *Visions of Rogers's science-based nursing: Unit 2: Practice.* (Publication No. 15-2285). New York: National League for Nursing.

Barrett, E. A. M. (Ed.). (1990b). *Visions of Rogers's science-based nursing: Unit 3: Research* (Publication No. 15-2285). New York: National League for Nursing.

Benedict, S. C., & Burge, J. M. (1990). The relationship between human field motion and preferred visible wavelengths. *Nursing Science Quarterly, 3,* 67-72.

Butcher, H. K., & Parker, N. I. (1988). Guided imagery within Rogers; science of unitary human beings: An experimental study. *Nursing Science Quarterly, 1,* 103-110.

Compton, M. A. (1989). A Rogerian view of drug abuse: Implications for nursing. *Nursing Science Quarterly, 2,* 98-105.

DeFeo, D. J. (1990). Change: A central concern of nursing. *Nursing Science Quarterly, 3,* 88-94.

Floyd, J. (1983). Research using Rogers' conceptual system: Development of a testable theorem. *Advances in Nursing Science, 5*(2), 37-48.

Girardin, B. (1990). *The relationship of light wave frequency and sleepwakefulness frequency in well, full-term Hispanic neonates.* Unpublished doctoral dissertation, Wayne State University, Detroit.

Heggie, J. R., Schoenmehl, P. A., Chang, M. K., & Grieco, C. (1989). Selection and implementation of Dr. Martha Rogers' nursing conceptual model in an acute care setting. *Clinical Nurse Specialist, 3,* 143-147.

Heidt, P. R. (1990). Openness: A qualitative analysis of nurses' and patients' experiences of therapeutic touch. *Image, 22,* 180-186.

Krieger, D. (1979). *The therapeutic touch: How to use your hands to help or heal.* Englewood Cliffs, NJ: Prentice-Hall.

Madrid, M., & Winstead-Fry, P. (1986). Rogers's conceptual model. In P. Winstead-Fry (Ed.), *Case studies in nursing theory* (pp. 73-102). New York: National League for Nursing.

Mason, T., & Patterson, R. (1990). A critical review of the use of Rogers' model within a special hospital: A single case study. *Journal of Advanced Nursing, 15,* 130-141.

Phillips, J. R. (1989). Science of unitary human beings: Changing research perspectives. *Nursing Science Quarterly, 2,* 57-60.

Quinn, J. F. (1989). Therapeutic touch as energy exchange: Replication and extension. *Nursing Science Quarterly, 2*(2), 79-87.

Schodt, C. M. (1989). Parental fetal attachment and couvade: A study of patterns of human-environment integrality. *Nursing Science Quarterly, 2,* 88-97.

Smith, M. C. (1988). Testing propositions derived from Rogers' conceptual system. *Nursing Science Quarterly, 1,* 60-67.

Smith, M. C. (1990). Pattern in nursing practice. *Nursing Science Quarterly, 3,* 57-59.

Wynd, C. A. (1990). Analysis of a power theory for health promotion activities. *Applied Nursing Research, 3,* 118-120.

Applications to Education

Barrett, E. A. M. (Ed.). (1990). *Visions of Rogers' science-based nursing: Unit 4: Education.* New York: National League for Nursing, Pub. No. 15-2285.

Rogers, M. E. (1985a). Nursing education: Preparation for the future. In *Patterns in education: The unfolding of nursing* (pp. 11-14). New York: National League for Nursing.

Rogers, M. E. (1985b). The nature and characteristics of professional education for nursing. *Journal of Professional Nursing, 1,* 381-383.

About the Author

Louette R. Johnson Lutjens, PhD, RN, is Associate Professor of nursing at Grand Valley State University in Allendale, Michigan. She received her Doctor of Philosophy in Nursing degree in 1990 from Wayne State University in Detroit, Michigan. Her research interests include nursing administrative issues related to nursing diagnosis, interventions, and aggregate patient outcomes and theory development and testing.